Emotional Wellness

The Other Half of Treating Cancer

For Rob & Charlene

To Many

Well Being Days!

Niki Barr

Emotional Wellness

The Other Half of Treating Cancer

by

Niki Barr, Ph.D.

Orion Wellspring, Inc.

Seattle

First edition, first printing March, 2013

Copyright © 2013 by Niki Barr, Ph.D., All rights reserved.

Published by Orion Wellspring, Inc., Seattle, WA 98109

(206) 931-4656

ISBN-13: 978-0615577463

ISBN-10: 0615577466

9 8 7 6 5 4 3 2 1

Printed and bound in the United States of America.

Orion Wellspring, Inc.

20 Blaine St.

Seattle, WA 98109

EMOTIONAL WELLNESS
The Other Half of Treating Cancer

CONTENTS

ACKNOWLEDGEMENTS

I wrote this book for, and dedicate it to, first my family members, some who lived and some who died with cancer, and then to those patients, family members, and caregivers who continued to "show up" for appointments, however difficult, to deal with numerous emotional challenges connected to the experience of living with cancer.

None of this could have come to fruition without Dr. Janice Tomberlin, Radiologist, who referred me to Valerie Oxford, MSSW (Master of Science in Social Work) at the University of Texas Southwestern Moncrief Cancer Institute. Keith Argenbright and Lori Drew, Medical Director and Executive Director respectively, along with staff members at the Institute, welcomed me to begin a pioneering psychotherapy practice working exclusively with cancer patients, their families, and their caregivers. Through Moncrief, I extended my practice to include The Center for

Cancer and Blood Disorders, Careity Foundation, Breast Care Center of North Texas, Texas Oncology, and Texas Health Harris Methodist Hospital in Fort Worth.

Additionally, many people continually inspired me to keep writing through to completion especially my cherished husband, Bob, my amazing children, my magnificent mom, and my dear friends, who I relied on and am most grateful for their belief in my oncology work and me. I would especially like to thank Orion Wellspring, Inc., for helping me publish this work. I relied on, and am most grateful for, their belief in my oncology work and me.

I am immensely blessed by each one of you. May Emotional *Wellness: The Other Half of Treating Cancer* be a gift back, in some way touching you and those you love and ever inspiring emotional wellness, whatever the circumstance.

~ Niki Barr, Ph.D.

FOREWORD

Through my experience working with cancer patients for several decades, I can tell you that creating a state of *wellbeing* is a vital part of the ability to survive. The sad part is that most of us do not learn about *survivor behavior* and how to maintain our wellbeing until our lives are threatened. Only then do we become enlightened; the "curse" becomes a blessing that we learn from and can share with others.

What I suggest is that we carefully review books already written, along with new ones like Dr. Barr's contribution, and use them all as resources to teach children how to deal with adversity and life's difficulties. If we start in childhood, we can ensure having *survivor behavior* as adults. All the sages of the past have told us how to accomplish this, but as life is now more technical and less personal, we need to use some current information to create a complete program encompassing mind, body and spirit.

One cannot really separate the three elements of mind, body, and spirit because our thoughts create our internal chemistry along with whatever spiritual beliefs and experiences influence our lives. Our bodies respond to the Body-Mind-Spirit Connection with the result of either disease or self-healing. To get the optimum result of healing, we have to understand and accept that our minds have that kind of power.

As a medical doctor, I described myself early on as a *tourist* in the world of diagnosis and disease because I had not lived what my patients were experiencing. However, after becoming a patient myself, I felt I had become a *native,* truly educated about a patient's *experience* of disease and not just the diagnosis.

This book will help you understand and treat your experience in a therapeutic way, and by that I do not mean just in terms of medical treatment to fight your disease—I mean marshaling all that is within you to add the *critical other half of healing* by using the Mind-Body-Spirit Connection successfully.

I saw the benefits of the lessons we can learn when my wife was diagnosed with a serious illness many years ago, and again just a few years ago. I was reminded of the terrible scare both she and I went through many years before her illness when our seven-year-old son's x-ray revealed a bone tumor. Apparently I was acting so out of character in his eyes as I tried to cope with this potentially devastating news that he was prompted to say, with that special wisdom children can display, "Dad, you're handling this poorly." I have since learned to "live the sermon, enjoy the day, and see the difference it makes in our lives and health."

For me accepting my mortality is an important component of what empowers me. By accepting that I have a limited time to live, I do not waste my life's time or let others make me unhappy. I control only one thing—my thoughts—and so death becomes my teacher about life. As Mother Teresa said, "I will not attend an anti-war rally, but if you ever have a peace rally, call me." So do not think of mortality as "the enemy" that you must fight, but instead expend your energy on loving your life and body and being well, physically and emotionally.

When you let your heart make up your mind you will make the right decisions. Your feelings and intuitive wisdom are vital in making the right choices. I use patients' dreams and drawings to help see what lies within us to empower our lives. This activity blocks the "rational brain's" tendency to allow the words of doctors to frighten us into thinking that, as the patient, we have no control over the outcome.

Wordswordswords can become *swordswordswords* but when **you** make the choices and not your doctor and family, you are choosing to go through the labor pains necessary for *self*-birthing. With this sense of control, you will undoubtedly have far fewer complications and side effects. Making the choice, guided by your intuition, is about deciding what is right for you and *not* about trying to avoid dying. We all die and so the key is living fully. Ask yourself what is accomplished by being bitter about everything you did or didn't do and then dying anyway?

Go ahead and have some of your "chocolate ice cream." I have letters from people who expected to die in a short time so went ahead and "lived" their chocolate ice cream. But they didn't die after all, and many end their letters with, "I didn't die and now I am so busy that I am *killing* myself! Help! Where do I go from here?" You take a nap…and then revisit the peaceful power of the Mind-Body-Spirit Connection.

There are qualities to the survivor personality that one can learn by reading this book and others. Absorb the wisdom of Dr. Barr and her recommendations of other authors who support her important work. We all can help you understand how to cope with a diagnosis of cancer and treatment—we are your support throughout the journey.

Please understand that you are not a statistic and you *do* have the potential to accomplish healing and wellbeing. It is not about miracles and spontaneous remissions. It is about self-induced healing through a state of wellbeing. Yes, this will require work on your part to control negative thoughts and to refocus on living by bringing faith, hope, humor and especially love into your life. It is not about failing—it is about *participating* in your life.

Your mind and body form a unit that is constantly interacting. I have had patients (who oncologists had little hope for) say they knew they would get well after I hugged them. Others responded to chemotherapy or radiation treatments that they believed in even when, due to technical errors, they were not actually receiving any. Still others had no side effects from their treatments because they told me, in effect, "I get out of the way and let it go to my tumor."

You are the key, living for yourself and living as your *authentic* self. This is not about being *selfish* but being *selfless.* Relationships keep us alive but it is a mistake to live *because* of them and die when they end. Live for yourself and the love you have to offer the world.

In the midst of difficulties, survivors are not afraid to express their feelings and shed tears. If you hide your feelings to protect others, you are hurting yourself and giving your body a mixed message. Share your needs and ask for help—that is *survival behavior*. When you are hungry you seek nourishment, so when dealing with emotions that are difficult for you to handle on your own *ask for emotional nourishment*. And when you need a hug ask for it!

Your emotions are stored in your body as is your childhood, so do not try to evade them. Confront what you need to let go of as well as what needs to be healed. When you suppress your anger to please others you are hurting yourself and your ability to heal; just as when you deny your depression and tell everyone you are fine. Survivors express their feelings and get the help they need. Anger is a motivating force, but turn its negative energy into the positive energy you need to recover in a healthy way. So let the charcoal and darkness of depression become a diamond and awaken you, lighting your path when you are under pressure.

Loneliness adversely affects your immune system's ability to function adequately, so find people and pets you can relate to. Statistics tell us that women live longer than men with the same cancers due to their relationships. While our mothers might be the first important *bond* we make in our life, the first and most important *relationship* we can form as we grow is a meaningful one with *ourselves.*

Before we can offer ourselves as loving people, good family members, friends, and co-workers, we have to find our *authentic* self within, and learn to really love that self. Yes, we can improve upon it as we learn the lessons of living, but we must nourish it with unconditional acceptance and love. It is then that all those with whom we interact will benefit the most from our presence in their lives.

So don't be "just Mom" and think life is over when the kids leave home. Don't be just "the wage earner" and give up because you can't work anymore. There is more to wellbeing than that. Rejoice in having that family or working relationship, but don't hang on because you feel empty inside, expecting others to feel responsible for your happiness. Instead, make it your life's work to give love. It comes back many-fold when it is given self**less**ly.

I want to include humor in this discussion of *survivor behavior.* A study revealed that cancer patients who laughed for no particular reason several times a day lived longer than the control group. We all have funny memories from the distant or more recent past, so think about them and laugh out loud every few hours. See how good it makes you feel. There are even Laughter Workshops and you may want to find one to experience the powerful healing of humor.

Survivor personalities reveal action, wisdom and devotion, so don't suffer as the submissive "good patient." Let this book help you to become a '**respant**,' or **res**ponsible partici***pant***. Ask for what you need to know from your doctors and make sure they ***stop, listen and answer you***. You are not a disease—you are a person and deserve to be treated like a person.

If you want to find a good doctor ask the doctor you are seeing now if she/he is ever criticized by patients, family members, and nurses. If they say "yes" then you can be assured you are working with a good doctor. A good doctor welcomes the chance to learn from patients and families, as well as from their own colleagues, about the mistakes they make. Good doctors do not blame the patient, but apologize and improve the way they practice medicine.

When I first started to submit articles to medical journals about my work with patients using the Mind-Body Connection, they sometimes came back saying, "Interesting but inappropriate for our journal." When I submitted the same articles to psychology journals for publication, they sometimes came back saying, "Appropriate but not interesting."

What I see as sad about the practice of medicine today is the focus on beliefs about treating disease that excludes an equal focus on the actual experiences of people living with the disease. In this book, Dr. Niki Barr shares the wisdom she has gained from counseling patients who are experiencing life with cancer. She gives patients tools to use for the other half of cancer treatment—emotional wellness. Experience teaches us what works and what is true, while beliefs can blind us to the truth.

So keep an open mind and work at loving your life and body so it gets this unmistakable message—"I am alive!" You do this by transforming your life, bringing order into it, and creating a sense of wellbeing.

In closing, please understand it is also vital to say "no" to the things you <u>do not</u> want to do. If you say "yes" to what others want of you, you are saying "no" to yourself, and that is not *survivor behavior*. It creates the opposite of wellbeing in your life and body.

Find your authentic self and *live your chocolate ice cream* by taking the time to eat, sleep, rest, play and laugh. When you do those things that make you lose track of time, you are living a creative and healthy life which will create wellbeing in your mind, body, and spirit.

If you have the inspiration and are willing to show up for practice, Dr. Niki Barr can be your coach and help you become a winner on this wondrous learning journey called Life.

- Bernie Siegel, MD

INTRODUCTION

Nothing can strike fear, anxiety, depression, grief, or overwhelm you more quickly than a cancer diagnosis. While medical advancements in the treatment of cancer continue to grow, concern with the *emotional wellness* of patients has been largely ignored as a vital part of cancer care until recently. Now, however, there is widespread agreement between both the medical community and the psychological community that healing is best served by tending to the physical *and* emotional needs of patients simultaneously.

It has been said that getting a cancer diagnosis "doesn't come with an instruction book." With *Emotional Wellness: The Other Half of Treating Cancer*, I hope to change that perception. This is a manual filled with simple, effective tools that strengthen emotional wellness at every step along the cancer journey from diagnosis through medical treatment, post treatment, and beyond.

This book is a "must have" for cancer patients, their family members, caregivers, friends, and coworkers. Each chapter gives clear and supportive ways for patients and everyone around them to express feelings and concerns as they arise during the healing journey. Addressing these emotions immediately is a vital part of strengthening emotional wellness.

The material for this book comes from my work with patients in all stages of cancer. Within the cancer resource center, I created a psychotherapy program for cancer patients who come in for one hour weekly sessions to explore and develop tools for coping with cancer. Family members and caregivers can join the patient in a session if the patient wishes, or can opt to have their own psychotherapy session. The people who come to see me are often scared, worried, tired, and uncertain about how to get themselves through cancer. Their loved ones are lost too, coping both with relationships, now centered on cancer, as well as their own concerns, fears, and worries.

Emotional Wellness: The Other Half of Treating Cancer is organized so that you can access tools that are appropriate to your stage of cancer treatment. Think about the image of a toolbox—an *emotional wellness toolbox*— into which you gather big and small tools which you know how to use when you need them. The book discusses aspects of living with cancer focusing on *emotional wellness* as a vital and constant companion on the journey.

The first three chapters provide you with ways to immediately turn your awakened emotions to your advantage and understand precisely how to express them to strengthen emotional wellness. You learn that emotional wellness is the *other half* of cancer treatment—there is *medical treatment* and its equal partner, *emotional wellness.*

A cancer diagnosis followed by medical treatment has been described as being in a blender whirling around with pieces of yourself flying everywhere. Your entire identity is shaken up. And if that weren't enough, the contents of the blender are continually changing depending on lab results, CT scans, how the medication is tolerated and many other variables.

Chapter One deals with the immediate aftermath of receiving a cancer diagnosis. Leading the emotional challenges early on is *Anxiety.* You will gain an understanding of your body's response to anxiety and why it is necessary to use tools to lessen those effects. The tools in this chapter are for use immediately and at any time anxiety threatens to overwhelm you.

Chapter Two describes medical treatment plans, moving *into the unknown* where procedures, scans, tests, and medications are prescribed by your doctor and carried out by your medical team. Depression can develop or deepen because therapies are physically taxing and disruptive to every aspect of your life—there is no more "normal." This chapter's list of tools, followed by a detailed "how to" for using them effectively, helps you cope with depression and strengthen your emotional wellness during the stress of treatment.

Chapter Three looks at what life is like after cancer. The outcome for many is that the experience of cancer is over—a once in a lifetime, albeit life changing, event. There is still, however, a need to strengthen and maintain emotional wellness. You will find emotional wellness tools to help you with issues like the changes in your body, your energy, your sex life, and your relationships. This chapter also includes ways to handle what is often uppermost in the minds of patients and those around them—the potential for recurrence and death.

Chapters Four, Five and Six cover negative outcomes that can occur following medical treatment. Our understanding of cancer and how to treat it effectively is still limited. Patients experience metastasis or recurrence with the worst case scenario being death. These outcomes cannot be ignored by patients and their families. Tools are needed to face them and ensure a better experience of life in the time that remains.

Whatever the medical treatment outcome life goes on, but cancer leaves an indelible mark on our lives. While everyone hopes, and some even predict, that life will return to how it once was, it will not.

Cancer calls you to meet it *head on* emotionally or be left in shambles. Choosing the path of emotional wellness allows you to face the physical and psychological demands of the cancer experience with a certain calm and confidence. You may want to enlist the help of an oncology social worker, psychologist, nurse, or psychotherapist for additional guidance and counseling.

Some patients I see express feelings of being both lost and at a loss. The experience of cancer creates such disorientation that they wonder "Who am I now?" Though cancer is sometimes described as a "dark night of the soul," many patients with the disease achieve emotional wellness as they develop a deeper understanding of themselves and discover a richer, more meaningful experience of life.

It is my hope that this book will be your ever-present and vital partner on the healing journey, helping you move through the life-changing cancer experience with emotional wellness.

1
A Cancer Diagnosis—
The Beginning

Anxiety is a feeling of fear, unease, and worry. In my practice, I see cancer patients whose anxiety is an "over the top" connection to life, a powerful energy often stemming from fearful thoughts, growing exponentially.

Anxiety clearly affects both cancer patients and their families. According to the National Cancer Institute (NCI), various aspects of the cancer journey are impacted by the ability to cope with anxiety such as keeping appointments, going through treatment, and the fear of recurrence. The NCI notes that, "Anxiety may increase pain, affect sleep, and cause nausea and vomiting. Even mild anxiety can affect the quality of life of patients with cancer and their families and may need to be treated." (NCI Adjustment to Cancer: Anxiety and Distress PDQ®)

Feeling anxious is a normal and emotionally healthy response to cancer. How could you not feel anxious? The key is to manage anxiety so it doesn't get out of hand. Review the tools list in the gray box below, followed by the detailed "How To" directions for using each of them.

TOOLS FOR ANXIETY

THE BASICS
Tangible items always available in your Emotional Wellness Toolbox include:
- This book
- A container to hold all of your materials
- Pen
- Pack of 3 x 5 index cards
- Spiral notebook
- Journal
- CDs—music
- CDs—meditation/relaxation; creative visualization; guided imagery

GIVE YOURSELF TIME
Put the brakes on temporarily

FIND OUT EVERYTHING YOU CAN
Making choices

KEEP A BINDER
Get all information organized

TRIANGLE BREATHING
Simple technique for immediate relief

'CATCH' ANXIOUS THOUGHTS
Stop the cycle of anxiety before it accelerates

MEDITATE
Learn to meditate and practice once a day

ERASE "WHAT IF" THINKING
Eliminate all "What If" self-talk completely

TWO EASY QUESTIONS TO STOP ANXIETY COLD
Ask yourself these questions right now

ONE QUESTION TO BRING CALM BACK
Ask yourself this question to soothe anxiety

FOCUS ON MAKING CHOICES
I am choosing to...

USING DISTRACTION
Specific tools for distracting yourself

GROUNDING YOURSELF
A simple strategy for eliminating anxiety Right Now!

GO FROM, "I CAN'T HANDLE THIS" to "I CAN HANDLE THIS!"
Learn to give yourself affirmation

ZOOM IN, ZOOM OUT
How to shift your focus from anxiety to a better feeling

YOUR FAVORITE MOVIE STAR
How she/he can help you with anxiety

HOW LONG CAN YOU 'BLANK' YOUR MIND
A game you can play for easing anxiety

LET IT GO, SHRED IT
A tool you can use this minute for anxiety relief

JOURNALING
Keep a journal to record your thoughts and feelings

REFUSE TO LISTEN TO CANCER 'HORROR STORIES'
Learn to tell people that their stories are harmful to your healing

'R E L A X' EXERCISE
How to calm yourself quickly with focus on breathing

LET THE PAPER HOLD IT
A tool for leaving anxiety behind

CHOOSING ONE
Apply problem solving technique to anxiety

DO THE OPPOSITE OF ANXIETY
Focusing on laughter

MAKE AN APPOINTMENT WITH A THERAPIST
Particularly, oncology trained, Very Helpful!

SUPPORT GROUPS
Try one or more to find support for relieving anxiety

FOCUS ON GOOD NUTRITION
Follow advice from doctor, nurse, and dietician

FOCUS ON PHYSICAL ACTIVITY
Include daily exercise prescribed and/or approved by your doctor

FOCUS ON RESTORATIVE SLEEP
Talk with your doctor for help with sleep problems

TOOLS - 'HOW TO'

GIVE YOURSELF TIME

When diagnosed with cancer alarm bells ring and you want to react—to do something or just *fix* this. But a quick reaction may not lead to the best treatment choices. It is better to give yourself time to sort out the diagnosis. Specifically, review what the doctor said, what the test results indicated, and what the initial treatment plan options are for you. Take a few days if you can—usually there is at least that much time—before any action on treatment is needed. Just sit with it alone, or talk about it, or if you journal regularly write about it. Use a method that is comfortable for you to arrive at an initial understanding of the diagnosis.

FIND OUT EVERYTHING YOU CAN

Once you have given yourself time to absorb the news of the diagnosis, write down a list of questions. Discuss these with at least one family member or friend and get their input. Schedule an appointment with your doctor to discuss treatment options. Even if they were discussed with you at diagnosis, you most probably could not "hear" them at that time. Go back in with a trusted family member or friend who will take notes as you ask your questions and learn specific information that you need.

KEEP A BINDER

You get a tremendous amount of information on treatment options, prescriptions, scans, reports, procedures, providers, and other resources. Start off immediately keeping a binder with tabs for every category. Keep this organized and handy so you can get to all of this important information quickly and easily. This binder is a very helpful tool to take with you each time you interact with various members of your medical team.

TRIANGLE BREATHING

Draw a triangle on a piece of paper in your spiral notebook. On the outer left side of the triangle, in the center of the line, write the letter I. On the outer right side of the triangle, in the center of the line, write the letter E. On the outer edge of the bottom, in the center of the line, write the letter P. I = Inhale, E = Exhale, and P = Pause.

Triangle breathing is a great tool for relaxation. You can learn it quickly and it can be used almost anywhere or anytime with the exception of when you are driving. The tool is most effective when it is used on a daily basis.

Take a deep breath in and then blow it out.

INHALE slowly while saying "inhale" silently.

EXHALE slowly while saying "exhale" silently.

PAUSE 1, 2, 3, 4 (you are not inhaling or exhaling now; if the pause feels too long, adjust the numbers as needed to feel comfortable).

Once you have tried the exercise several times you can substitute a favorite word, phrase, or color for the word "pause" and for the counted numbers. For example, inhale slowly, exhale slowly, and then say PEACE or CALM or BLUE. Drag these words out to a count of 4 to get your full pause, or whatever is comfortable. Using this tool with a meaningful word, color, or phrase enhances relaxation.

You may decide to have several different words or phrases to use for specific situations. When you are going to see your doctor, perhaps the word "relax" is effective for you. When you are going back to work, you could use the phrase "I am calm and confident." Once you've tried the exercise several times, you can substitute a favorite word, phrase, or color for the word pause and for the counted numbers. For example, inhale slowly, exhale slowly then say PEACE or CALM or

BLUE. Drag these words out to a count of 4 to get your full pause, or whatever is comfortable. Choose a meaningful word, color, or phrase that enhances relaxation.

Work with triangle breathing before you need it, as it is a skill requiring practice to be effective.

CATCHING ANXIOUS THOUGHTS

Anxious thoughts are thought over and over again resulting in anxiety. The trick to dealing with anxiety is to catch anxious feelings before they intensify. Slow down and think through what you are telling yourself about the situation at hand.

Write your thoughts down on a note card, one thought per card. See if you can identify what ONE thought that started the chain reaction resulting in your feeling anxious. Then identify the second thought coming after the first thought. Continue in this manner, thought after thought, in order.

Now, start with the initial thought leading to feeling anxiety and write down a new thought which does *not* result in feeling anxiety. What new thought could you substitute for the first old anxious thought? The new thought is confident and empowering. Continue down the line of thoughts until you have completed your list.

MEDITATION

Many CD's are available to help learn how to meditate or for providing guided imagery for meditation.

Try:

How to Meditate with Pema Chodron: A Practical Guide to Making Friends with Your Mind.

or

Meditation for Beginners by Jack Kornfield

or

Guided Mindfulness Meditation by Jon Kabat-Zin

Please see RESOURCES at the end of the book for more tools.

ERASE "WHAT IF" THINKING

Refuse to play the "What If?" game.

What if the cancer has spread? What if medical treatment doesn't work? What if I can't take care of her? What if he dies?

One *What If* question leads to another and then another, often spiraling into anxiety. Awareness is the way to stop yourself immediately when you start asking *What If?* questions. Instead, ask yourself the two questions in the next tool.

TWO EASY QUESTIONS TO STOP ANXIETY COLD

Is this thought helping me or hurting me?

Is this thought moving me forward or moving me backward?

BRINGING "CALM" BACK

Soothe yourself in the moment. What would feel especially good right now… a cup of tea, another pillow, listening to some music?

FOCUS ON MAKING CHOICES

"I am choosing to….." Choosing is active and empowering. Make a conscious decision to substitute "I am choosing to" for "I have to, I don't want to, I must".

USING DISTRACTION

Work with this tool BEFORE you need it. Choose a favorite place, at the beach, in the library, taking a drive in the country, etc. Think of everything you can about this scene including colors, smells, people involved, sounds, tastes, and how it feels when you're there. Build it up very clearly in your mind, going over and over it, so when you want to use the "distraction" tool you can recall both where it is and tiny details about it. You might want to come up with two or three of these scenarios.

Use this when you're waiting for a medical procedure, getting a medical procedure, you're waiting for the one you love getting a medical procedure, or whenever it would be useful for you.

GROUNDING YOURSELF

Stop anxious thoughts in their tracks, by "grounding" yourself or focusing on details. The room you are in right now, what color is the carpet, the wall, what pictures are hanging on the walls, what color is the table, the chairs. What do the light fixtures look like; do you see dust on them? The person talking to you, what color are her/his eyes, her/ his hair, what is she/he wearing? Being very focused on another set of thoughts *interrupts* a chain of anxious thoughts.

MOVE FROM, "I CAN'T HANDLE THIS"

Yes, you CAN handle whatever is going on five minutes at a time. You can do anything five minutes at a time.

Remind yourself you CAN get through the next five minutes and the next five minutes after that. Soon you will look back and notice you got through a bunch of five-minute time blocks.

ZOOM IN, ZOOM OUT

Think of a camera. You can zoom in for a close-up or you can take a regular picture. Using the same idea, you can check in with yourself to see how things are going by zooming in. Ask yourself how am I feeling; how are things going in my world; how am I in my immediate surroundings? Then, zoom out and ask yourself, "How am I in the big picture in relation to family members and friends; my community; life in general?" Using Zoom In/Zoom Out gives you a quick reading of how things are going *from a balanced perspective*. You can then ask yourself if any adjustments need to be made up close *and* evaluate how you are doing "in the big picture."

With anxiety, zooming out in particular provides relief. Since anxiety tends to be focused on what's in your immediate, "up close" attention, choosing to pull back (zoom out) brings perspective and balance. That perspective becomes clear by supportive self talk like, "I'm not the *only* one who has gone through this." It may help divert you to problem-solving mode and away from anxiety by asking yourself, "I wonder if I could find resources in places I haven't even thought of so far?"

YOUR FAVORITE MOVIE STAR

Choose a movie star you admire, one who is calm and confident. Imagine how that movie star would handle the situation you are in. What would she/he say to the doctor, to the friend who is offering endless advice, to the insurance company? You've probably heard the saying "fake it til' you make it." Put on you "calm and confident" self to manage anxiety.

HOW LONG CAN YOU BLANK YOUR MIND?

See how long you can blank your mind, not thinking any thought. Can you do it for five seconds… ten seconds…longer?   Sometimes it's helpful to let your mind rest. Cancer brings with it many and varied things to deal with medically, emotionally, and within relationships. Taking a "thought break" can bring much needed respite, if only for a few seconds at a time. The more you use this tool, the longer you can sustain the "thought break."

LET IT GO, SHRED IT

In her book *The Artist's Way*, Leslie Cameron describes an exercise of writing three pages of thoughts and feelings each morning before you do anything else. This is an excellent tool for "dumping out" thoughts and feelings.

Many people I work with are very hesitant to use this tool because of concerns that someone will find and read what they write down. To alleviate this concern, I suggest shredding the pages after completing them. The tool becomes even more powerful when focusing on "letting go" of troublesome thoughts and feelings as the papers are shredded.

JOURNAL

Journaling on the other hand, is a progression of thoughts and feelings you write down as desired. Some people find re-reading what they have written very helpful.

A related tool is the video journal. If you have a newer model computer, the camera is built in. You can film yourself discussing thoughts and feelings.

REFUSE TO LISTEN TO CANCER "HORROR" STORIES

Stop listening to cancer "horror stories." Everyone has them and everyone seems ready to tell them without thinking how these stories might affect the listener. When someone starts telling you one of them, let the speaker know that you prefer <u>not</u> to hear it, then change the subject.

R-E- L-A-X Exercise

Find a quiet place without distractions. After taking a few slow breaths, inhale while saying "R." Then, exhale while saying "E." Continue in this way spelling the word "RELAX," one letter for each inhale, and one letter for each exhale.

CHOOSING ONE

Make a list of your concerns in your spiral notebook. Choose one of them and write it down on a note card. What one thing, only ONE thing could you DO to ease your concern. Then, DO it.

DO THE OPPOSITE OF ANXIETY

What's funny for you? What makes you laugh? Get a joke book, spend time with a friend who *cracks you up*, watch a movie that makes you giggle, or recall a memory that makes you laugh every time you think about it.

MAKE AN APPOINTMENT WITH A THERAPIST

Think of making an appointment with a therapist as a gift to yourself. A therapist, particularly one who has oncology training, can help you navigate the experience of cancer from diagnosis on, keeping you focused throughout on emotional wellness.

SUPPORT GROUPS

Support groups can be wonderful for providing both information and emotional support. Some people hesitate to go to these, but before you dismiss this option, at least check several out to see how a group could benefit you.

FOCUS ON GOOD NUTRITION

Eat well. Consult your doctor about what foods will be best. Some treatment centers or resource centers have dieticians who will provide important nutritional information for your diet as a cancer patient.

FOCUS ON PHYSICAL ACTIVITY

After discussing physical activity with your doctor, carry out what is permissible. Some of my patients choose not to take advantage of being cleared by their doctors to walk around the block or participate in an exercise class designed for cancer patients. I remind them that studies continue to be published saying exercise helps people feel better both physically and emotionally.

FOCUS ON RESTORATIVE SLEEP

Many CD's or MP3 downloads are on the market to help with sleep.

Try:

Sleep Through Insomnia by KRS Edstrom

or

Just Relax- Relaxing to Sleep CD, by Gail Seymour

Please see RESOURCES at the end of this book for additional suggestions about getting more restorative sleep.

SUMMARY

A cancer diagnosis brings with it an unforgettable emotional "slam." Anxiety often kicks in as you wonder what will happen to you and to your family members. It is a normal emotional response to feel anxious when you have a cancer diagnosis or in the support circle of someone who does. The key to effectively coping with anxiety is learning how to manage it through your breathing and both written and oral self talk.

2
Into the Unknown—Medical Treatment

Depression and cancer are often linked. Feelings of sadness and despair are not uncommon, wherever in the cancer journey you may be. If depression interferes with daily functioning and has lasted two successive weeks, talk with your doctor. Guidelines suggest depression lasting two successive weeks is *clinical depression* and is widely regarded by the medical community to be treatable through medication and/or counseling. Approximately 25% of cancer patients are clinically depressed.

Signs to look for include:

- Loss of interest in daily activities
- Persistent sadness or feeling of emptiness
- Sleep disturbances
- Significant weight loss or gain

- Loss of concentration

- Fatigue

- Suicidal thoughts or behavior

The National Cancer Institute, American Cancer Society, and the Mayo Clinic (Ness, 2010) note that sometimes it is difficult to determine if symptoms of depression are coming from cancer (e.g., loss of appetite related to medicine, insomnia related to medicine) or are, in fact, the result of clinical depression.

In my psychotherapy work with cancer patients, I often defined depression as a "disconnect from life." Think about depressed people you may have encountered. This person has little energy for anything. She/he is sad, tired, hopeless, feels miserable, and in a funk.

Once you understand what depression is, the key is to do something about it. Talk with your doctor, and / or schedule an appointment with a social worker or a psychologist. This is an important step to take in order to move forward.

TOOLS FOR DEPRESSION

THE BASICS
Tangible items always available in your Emotional Wellness
Toolbox
- This book
- A container to hold all of your materials
- Pen
- Pack of 3 x 5 index cards
- Spiral notebook
- Journal
- CDs—music
- CDs—meditation/relaxation; creative visualization;
  guided imagery

MEDICAL CARE
Meeting roller coaster emotions head on

KEEP A ROUTINE
Taking care of you

EMPOWERING RELATIONSHIPS
Taking a break from "cancer talk"

THE WORLD JUST GOES ON
Feeling alone

THREE THINGS YOU CAN DO RIGHT NOW
Simple technique for easing depression

YOUR OWN AFFIRMATIONS
Creating true statements for moving yourself forward

MOVE YOURSELF FORWARD ONE NUMBER AT A TIME
Easy tool for feeling better immediately

TIMING OUT
Interrupting depression, moving forward

WHAT WOULD A MENTOR OR A WISE SAGE
ADVISE ME TO DO?
Thinking through what she/he would recommend

WHAT'S KEEPING ME STUCK?
How to get "unstuck" from depression

WHAT COULD I DO FOR ME RIGHT NOW?
Taking care to take care of you

ENCOURAGING YOURSELF WITH SELF TALK
Have a conversation with yourself

MAKE ONE "ME" GOAL EVERY SINGLE DAY
The power of one daily goal

ONE HAPPY THOUGHT CAN BE IMPACTFUL
Simple and effective tool for changing depression

JOURNAL YOUR FEELINGS AND THOUGHTS
Writing your feelings on paper brings relief

MAKE AN APPOINTMENT WITH A SOCIAL WORKER OR
PSYCHOLOGIST
Helpful for navigating cancer

SUPPORT GROUPS
Beneficial for offering support and information

PHYSICAL EXERCISE
Ask your doctor what you can do for exercise during medical
care.

FOCUS ON GOOD NUTRITION
Follow advice from doctor, dietician

FOCUS ON PHYSICAL ACTIVITY
Include daily exercise your doctor has prescribed

FOCUS ON RESTORATIVE SLEEP
Talk with your doctor about ways to improve your sleep (see the resources in Appendix A of this book)

TOOLS 'HOW TO'

MEDICAL CARE, UPS AND DOWNS

Expect many emotional "ups and downs" during your medical care. Your doctor and medical team are focused on treating cancer using the best information available. Changes are made within treatment plans based on how you are responding. Depending on what is included in your treatment plan, changes can be made in chemotherapy type and dosing schedule, radiation therapy type and dosing schedule, surgical intervention, prescription medications, and any other diagnostic or treatment modalities. These changes can "rock" emotions with highs and lows and everything in between.

Put your focus on "right now." Keep thinking in the *present moment.* Tell yourself that "…right now, in the treatment plan, we are…" Don't pile on the potential problems of treatment plan changes before they happen.

When a change is made, then at that point you can tell yourself, "…with this change in the treatment plan, we are now…" and avoid the "What If?" trap entirely. Feel what you feel *in the moment* as you move through the treatment plan. Your emotions are responses to what is happening and are very normal. It is **not** normal when your emotional responses interfere with the activities of daily life. If you cannot function in any area of your daily life because emotions are out of control, it is important to talk with your doctor.

KEEP A ROUTINE

Medical care brings much change into your life. In my experience as a psychotherapist in the field of oncology, I have learned from cancer patients how important daily routines are to "feeling better." Try to schedule appointments at the same time during the day. Try to wake up and go to sleep at the same time each morning and evening. Try to eat each meal at the same time every day. All of these routines are important but often very challenging for cancer patients. Try to establish at least one or two of these routines as early in your healing journey as you can, but always be kind and gentle with yourself—tell yourself that you will do these helpful things when you are able.

EMPOWERING RELATIONSHIPS

Relationships are vital for emotional wellness. Cancer can ignite emotions in patients and their loved ones and spill over from one relationship to another. Not surprisingly, cancer very often takes center stage within relationships crowding out time to focus on anything else.

It's okay to take a break from talking about cancer. In fact, decide on some "rules" regarding "cancer-talk" by saying something like:

"We will talk about cancer for 15 minutes after the kids go to bed, then we will focus on other things."

"Mom, thank you for your care and concern. This is what's going on…" [summarize your information about cancer] then go on to say, *"I'd like to spend the rest of our time talking about other things."*

THE WORLD JUST GOES ON

While you have people around you who care and love you, their lives do go on. As you observe that people are carrying on with their lives, you are focused on having a cancer diagnosis, coping with medical care, and whatever else is to come. A deep sense of aloneness can result. It's a normal feeling. Talk about it, journal about it, and allow yourself to feel what you feel. Emotional wellness comes from opening doors in your heart and mind—letting light shine in. It is compromised by repressing your feelings because you think somehow they are "bad" or otherwise negative. The energy you need now more than ever comes from strengthening emotional wellness.

THREE THINGS YOU *CAN* DO

On one of the 3 x 5 index cards you should always have handy, list three things you truly enjoy doing. Are you currently doing any of these? If you are, skip this tool.

If you aren't, why aren't you? Is it because you don't make time to include at least one of these favorite activities? Is it because you can no longer do them due to cancer-based changes? Staying connected and doing what you love is very important for emotional wellness. Brainstorm how to modify each activity you've listed on your note card as needed.

Sample modifications of activities:

Can't garden? Sit in your garden.

Can't be outside? Put your chair by the window, watch the birds, look at the flowers, make cloud pictures. Or, look at books filled with nature pictures, watch a nature program on TV, draw a garden.

Can't focus on reading? Listen to a book on tape found at your library, at the bookstore, or online. Flip through a magazine. Perhaps focusing on a short article will be more satisfying than trying to read a book right now.

Can't fish? Watch fishing shows on TV; read fishing magazines.

Can't cook? Look at recipes, cooking magazines, recipes online.

Can't dance? Watch the dancing shows on TV. Rent a dancing movie.

Can't build projects? Read about project for building later.

Make a plan to do what you enjoy

Decide what time of the day you will do one of these activities

Lay out what you will do

If it's painting a picture, set your paints, brushes, and canvas out, ready to go.

If it's knitting a scarf, lay your needles, yarn, and pattern out, ready to go.

If it's a wood working TV show, let your family members know you will be watching it at 4:00 p.m.

Follow through

DO the thing(s) you enjoy as planned. This is your "connect back up" tool. Depressed people tend <u>not</u> to follow through. Don't make this mistake. *A key element of dealing with depression is taking action.*

YOUR OWN AFFIRMATIONS

On a 3 x 5 card write down an affirmation you find encouraging, inspiring, or helpful. This affirmation may be a quote from a famous person, a Bible verse, or one you create. Read this affirmation often, keeping it with you.

A variety of affirmations may be beneficial depending on what you're dealing with at the present time. Each time you find one you like write it down on a 3 x 5 card. Soon you will have a stack of cards with affirmations to be used as needed.

MOVE YOURSELF FORWARD ONE NUMBER AT A TIME

Ask yourself what number you are right now on a scale from 1-10, #1 being not depressed at all and #10 being very depressed. If you are very depressed, call your doctor. If you are somewhat depressed, see if you can decrease your number by taking some kind of action. Turn it into a game. "I wonder if I could move from #5 to #4?" "What could I do to feel a little better?" Then, see if you can move yourself down another number.

Write down in your spiral notebook what actions you take that are helpful for you. Use this as a tool for decreasing depression as needed.

TIMING OUT

Set a timer for 15 minutes, 30 minutes, an hour or whatever amount of time feels comfortable for giving yourself a break, then use this time as a "time out." Read a magazine, watch a movie, listen to some music, take a shower, pet the dog, go for a walk, sit in the backyard, or do whatever will use the time you have set for your break.

The only rule that goes with this tool is doing something pleasurable just for you. The result of doing something pleasurable just for you is relaxation. This time out gives you time away from depression. Just for a little while you are setting depression aside.

WHAT WOULD A MENTOR OR A WISE SAGE ADVISE ME TO DO?

Choose a person you know and truly admire or choose someone you would like to know who has admirable characteristics. What do you think this person would advise you to do if they were in your situation?

This is a good tool for brainstorming ways to handle or cope with depression, other emotions, and various situations. Keep a list of these ideas in your spiral notebook for reference.

WHAT'S KEEPING ME STUCK?

Sometimes you can find yourself psychologically "stuck," similar to having one foot on the accelerator and the other on the brake at the same time.

Write down in your spiral notebook the following:

What do I think is keeping me stuck?

Do I want more information? If so, what kind of information?

Do I want to make a decision? If so, what is the decision?

Do I want help with some part? If so, what kind of help? Who can help?

Do I need to take action? What action?

What other questions would be helpful to ask yourself?

Simply identifying how you are stuck and problem solving how you can get unstuck can be particularly beneficial. Take time for getting your thoughts on paper about being stuck. Then, move forward.

WHAT COULD I DO FOR ME RIGHT NOW?

When you take time to ask yourself this question, you will usually get an answer. Maybe you'd like to call a friend, have a cup of coffee, power nap, or listen to some music.

This tool often gets ignored when you're "caught up" with medical care and the demands of daily life. However, asking the question and following through can provide surprising and very beneficial results.

ENCOURAGING YOURSELF WITH SELF-TALK

Connect back up with yourself through compassion. You could say something like:

"It's okay to feel what I feel. Having cancer isn't an easy thing to go through. Medical care for cancer involves a lot of time and energy and it is affecting my relationships. I have a lot on my plate right now. "

Continue with this conversation, talking to yourself in a kind and supportive way. Go ahead and speak aloud when you are by yourself to boost the effectiveness of this tool.

MAKE ONE "ME" GOAL EVERY SINGLE DAY

Each day decide on one goal you will accomplish for yourself. It can be as simple as taking out the trash, reading the newspaper, checking e-mail, or running an errand.

Write your goal on a 3 x 5 card and keep it with you. When you have reached the goal, write down a new goal for the next day. Then file the one you just reached. Watching these cards pile up is evidence of achievement and a successful connection with yourself.

ONE HAPPY THOUGHT CAN BE IMPACTFUL

What one happy thought could you think about? This tool requires only one. Find one happy thought you can bring to your mind throughout the day.

JOURNAL YOUR FEELINGS AND THOUGHTS

A journal provides a place for emptying your feelings and thoughts. Writing these down as often as you like often brings relief, understanding, and insight into whatever you are experiencing.

A variation of the written journal is to journal through video. Newer model computers have cameras built in or you could set up a video camera.

MAKE AN APPOINTMENT WITH A SOCIAL WORKER OR PSYCHOLOGIST

Oncology trained therapists understand cancer and emotions. Use this resource for navigating through cancer.

SUPPORT GROUPS

Ask your doctor and medical team for information about support groups in your community. See how one or more could be helpful for you, providing both support and information.

PHYSICAL EXERCISE

After discussing physical activity with your doctor, carry out what is permissible. Some of my patients choose not to take advantage of being cleared by their doctors to walk around the block or participate in an exercise class designed for cancer patients. I remind them that studies continue to be published saying exercise helps people feel better both physically and emotionally.

FOCUS ON GOOD NUTRITION

Follow advice from your doctor. Sometimes even when you can eat certain foods, they don't taste good.

Experimentation and creativity will help, including talking with a dietician on staff.

FOCUS ON PHYSICAL ACTIVITY

Your doctor will give you guidelines for getting exercise. Be sure to follow through on what is recommended, as exercise is very helpful with managing depression.

FOCUS ON RESTORATIVE SLEEP

Talk with your doctor if you are having trouble with sleep. It is not unusual for sleep patterns to be interrupted during medical care. Please see RESOURCES in the back of this book for helpful CD's and other information.

SUMMARY

Depression is a normal emotional response to having cancer. If you have depression lasting more than two weeks and depression is interfering with your activities of daily life, it is very important to talk with your doctor. When you feel depressed, or "disconnected" from daily living, it is essential to "connect back up" through a variety of ways including medication, counseling, and specific emotional wellness tools.

You may use any or all of these for moving through depression.

3
Outcomes—Post Medical Treatment

Hearing the words, "Come back for a follow up visit in X months…" and "You are finished with treatment…" at your last doctor visit is cause for great celebration. But after the celebration, perhaps within a few days, a week, a month or even longer it is not uncommon for me to see patients who express thoughts about the difficulty of rejoining "regular" life. Life during cancer was centered on daily and /or weekly medical appointments, medical procedures, and "built up" relationships with members of their medical care team. . Suddenly, after dreaming of the day it would all be finished, they find themselves asking, "Now, it's all over?" Some patients feel as though they've been dropped off at the curb and are unsure about what to do now.

A cancer patient's life necessarily centers on the disease and treatment. Now that is over. How can patients merge back into regular life? Experiencing life without cancer brings with it other emotional vulnerabilities. Think of the multi-faceted dimensions you are dealing with or have dealt with throughout diagnosis and treatment. These may include: body parts that have been removed or significantly changed, "chemo brain," sexual concerns, physical energy level, religious and spiritual beliefs, relationships, and whether to return to work.

Additionally, fear of recurring cancer tends to gather momentum as you return for follow-up doctor visits. It is not uncommon to find yourself worried when you notice a pain here or a pain there in your body, wondering if the cancer has come back or spread to another place.

Emotional reactions in this post-cancer period, with its challenge of rejoining daily life, tend to move between anxiety and depression. What you are feeling *is normal* given all you have experienced between diagnosis and medical care. If you find your emotions are interfering with activities of daily life, please contact your doctor.

TOOLS FOR ANXIETY & DEPRESSION

The Basics: Tangible items always available in your Emotional Wellness Toolbox
- This book
- A container to hold all of your materials
- Pen
- Pack of 3 x 5 index cards
- Spiral notebook
- Journal
- CDs—music
- CDs—meditation/relaxation; creative visualization; guided imagery

BINDER CHECK AND NEW TAB
Make certain all papers from treatment are filed, new tab for follow up visits

ESTABLISH DAILY ROUTINE POST MEDICAL CARE
Moving forward into daily life

FOCUS ON MAKING CHOICES
You decide....

MOVING FORWARD NUMBER BY NUMBER
Easing emotion

A QUESTION YOU DON'T ALLOW YOURSELF
Don't Entertain This One

MEDITATION
Letting go, mindfulness

WHAT COULD I DO FOR ME RIGHT NOW?
Taking care of my needs/wants

TRIANGLE BREATHING
It's all in the pause

THINK ONE HAPPY THOUGHT
Simple tool for moving forward

SELF-TALK TAKES YOU THROUGH
Be your own coach

CANCER STORIES BE GONE!
The power of changing the subject

BREATHING STRATEGY
Using a "RELAX" tool

THE JOURNAL OR SHRED IT
Expressing feelings and thoughts

SHIFTING YOUR FOCUS
Zooming in and zooming out

PROBLEM SOLVING ONE ISSUE
No "megasizing" this tool

I CAN HANDLE THIS
What you tell yourself matters

COUNSELING
Psychotherapy, post-medical care

SUPPORT GROUP
Offers both support and information focused on post medical care

EATING
Changing tastes, favorite foods?

EXERCISE
Actively participating for physical and emotional health

SLEEPING
Talk with your doctor about ways to improve your sleep

TOOLS 'HOW TO'

BINDER CHECK AND NEW TAB

Check to be sure all papers are organized and filed in your binder that may be left over from medical care.

Make a new **Post-Medical Care** tab for your binder. While you won't have the volume of papers to file as you did during medical care, you will have follow-up visits and miscellaneous papers.

ESTABLISH NEW ROUTINE POST- MEDICAL CARE

To make it easier to rejoin daily life, form a new routine for yourself. Since you no longer have various medical appointments, what makes sense for your daily schedule now? Going back to work? Working at home? Continuing to stay at home as you did pre-cancer? Among patients I have seen, it is not uncommon to develop a "lost feeling" when a new daily structure isn't established.

FOCUS ON MAKING CHOICES

During medical care, you don't have as much freedom to make choices since the doctor is only available during certain times, chemotherapy/radiation can only be scheduled at certain times, and scans or other medical tests can only be scheduled at specified times. Within those parameters, you really had no choice but to live by the schedule dictated by the availability of the medical care team. Various degrees of anxiety and depression can result from no longer having that structure.

Now, you are actively focusing on making new choices as you rejoin regular daily life. Using the words, "I am choosing to…" empowers you and stimulates emotional wellness in this post-treatment chapter of your life.

MOVING FORWARD NUMBER BY NUMBER

Play the "Where am I on the one to ten scale?" game again. With #1 being "very little of the emotion" and #10 being "intense emotion," what number describes how you feel? See if you can lower the number with a specific tool described earlier, like Triangle Breathing, Journaling, or Meditating.

As always, call your doctor if your emotions are interfering with functioning in your activities of daily life.

A QUESTION YOU DON'T ALLOW YOURSELF

Do not entertain the question "What if?" What if's can create emotional upheaval very quickly.

What if this pain I feel in my arm means cancer is coming back?

What if the cancer returns and spreads?

What if I have to have more surgery/chemo/radiation?

What if, what if, what if, what if, what if?

If you've played the "what if" game, you know just one "what if" leads to countless others. Choose <u>not</u> to begin playing the game, or if you find yourself playing, STOP.

MEDITATION

Mindfulness meditation is a tool to help you stay focused in the present, "the right now." It is very effective for helping you relax by teaching you how to eliminate anxious, shallow breathing. Many instructional CD's are available for learning how to meditate, for advanced meditation, and for guided imagery.

Please see RESOURCES at the end of the book for CD's and other materials.

WHAT COULD I DO FOR ME RIGHT NOW?

Frequently, throughout the day, ask yourself what one thing you could do right now for yourself. Would you like to have a cup of soup, take a power nap, get a glass of water, or do something else? While this is a simple tool it is surprisingly powerful for enhancing emotional wellness.

TRIANGLE BREATHING

Triangle breathing is a great tool for relaxation. You can learn it quickly and it can be used almost anywhere or anytime with the exception of when you are driving. The tool is most effective when it is used on a daily basis.

Draw a triangle on a piece of paper in your spiral notebook. On the outer left side of the triangle, in the center of the line, write the letter I. On the outer right side of the triangle, in the center of the line, write the letter E. On the outer edge of the bottom, in the center of the line, write the letter P. I = Inhale, E = Exhale, and P = Pause.

Take a deep breath in and then blow it out.

INHALE slowly while saying "inhale" silently.

EXHALE slowly while saying "exhale" silently.

PAUSE 1, 2, 3, 4 (you are not inhaling or exhaling now; if the pause feels too long, adjust the numbers as needed to feel comfortable).

Once you have tried the exercise several times you can substitute a favorite word, phrase, or color for the word "pause" and for the counted numbers. For example, inhale slowly, exhale slowly, and then say **PEACE or CALM or BLUE.** Drag these words out to a count of four to get your full pause, or whatever is comfortable. Using this tool with a meaningful word, color, or phrase enhances relaxation.

You may decide to have several different words or phrases to use for specific situations. When you are going to see your doctor, perhaps the word "relax" is effective for you. When you are going back to work, you could use the phrase "I am calm and confident."

THINK ONE HAPPY THOUGHT

What one happy thought could you think about right now, just one?

You might want to start a list of happy thoughts in your spiral notebook. Continue adding to your list as these thoughts come to you. When you're having a particularly hard day, write down one of the happy thoughts on a 3 x 5 card, taking it with you and referring to it often throughout the day.

SELF-TALK TAKES YOU THROUGH

Be your own coach. Talk yourself gently through a situation, one step at a time similar to moving forward segment by segment (see tool Getting through a Challenging Time described in Chapter 4).

Or, you could imagine someone coming to you looking for advice about the same situation and ask yourself, "How would I coach this person?"

CANCER STORIES BE GONE!

Changing the subject is top priority when your Aunt Sue, your dad, or your friend's friend, want to tell you cancer stories. Their stories are usually about how someone they know, or someone they just know of, had the same cancer as you, and they color the story with dramatic details of recurrence and other negative outcomes. This is not helpful for you. While you may not "take in" the story, little strands of fear can start growing and escalating. If the conversation is headed in that direction, head it off by saying you'd rather not hear the story. Be firm and quickly ask, "What else can we talk about?"

CHANGE YOUR BREATHING, INCREASE YOUR RELAXATION

Find a quiet place without distractions. After taking a few slow breaths, inhale while saying "R." Then, exhale while saying "E." Continue in this way spelling the word "RELAX" using one letter for each inhale, and one letter for each exhale.

You could use this same tool with other words such as "calm" or "peace."

THE JOURNAL OR SHRED IT

Cancer patients I work with seem evenly divided on which of these tools they think are most beneficial. On the one hand, pouring thoughts and feelings out on journal pages, reading and re-reading them, and adding quotes or insights reportedly result in a cathartic release. Research indicates this is a very effective tool for that purpose.

On the other hand, some patients feel very guarded and cautious often choosing not to use a journal fearing others will read what they wrote down. Their concern outweighs the benefit of journaling. Instead they choose to write down their thoughts and feelings and then take the pages to the shredder or use scissors to manually shred the pages. This tool provides both the cathartic benefits of getting thoughts and feelings out and the need to protect the process from other eyes by shredding the pages when finished. You, too, may find using a combination of journaling and shredding works best to allay any fear about others reading what you have written.

SHIFTING YOUR FOCUS WITH ZOOMING

Think of a camera. You can zoom in for a close-up or you can take a regular picture. Using the same idea, you can check in with yourself to see how things are going by zooming in. Ask yourself how am I feeling; how are things going in my world; how am I in my immediate surroundings? Then, zoom out and ask yourself, "How am I doing *in the big picture* with family members and friends, my community, and life in general?" Using Zoom In/Zoom Out gives you a quick reading of how things are going from a balanced perspective. You can then ask yourself if any adjustments need to be made up close and evaluate how you are doing *in the big picture.*

With anxiety, zooming out in particular provides relief. Since anxiety tends to be focused on what's in your immediate, *up close* attention, choosing to *pull back* (zoom out) brings perspective and balance. That perspective becomes clear by supportive self-talk like, "I'm not the only one who has gone through this." It may help divert you to problem-solving mode and away from anxiety by asking yourself, "I wonder if I could find resources in places I haven't even thought of so far?"

With depression as with anxiety, zooming out is very effective. Like anxiety, depression finds you caught up in the immediate focus of "my sadness" and "my feeling of being disconnected from life." You can get so focused on your own picture (zoomed in) that you forget that life outside of your *up close* world offers quite a lot. *Pulling back* (zooming out) allows you to begin reconnecting with life and helps you see the bigger picture where other people with concerns are still having fun as active participants in life.

PROBLEM-SOLVING ONLY ONE ISSUE

There is no need to "megasize" this tool. What ONE thing could you do *right now* to problem-solve whatever is bothering you?

First, write the problem down at the top of a page in your spiral notebook. Then write down any and every solution you can think of. When your list of solutions is finished, select something on the list that you **can do right now** to solve, or at least begin to solve, what's bothering you. Continue taking action until the problem is solved. Tackling one problem at a time gives you a sense of accomplishment that isn't available if you are overwhelmed and scattered in your problem-solving efforts. This tool will empower you and produce significant self-confidence!

I CAN HANDLE THIS

What you tell yourself matters. If your thoughts are centered on "I can't handle this" self-talk, or if you continually use the "I can't handle this" phrase in talking with your family and friends, you are setting up a self-fulfilling prophecy. You start really believing you, in fact, can't handle the situation. But you are telling yourself a lie.

You CAN move through whatever is going on *for five minutes at a time*. Use self-talk like, "Of course I can handle this for five minutes at a time." Take action and move forward in this manner.

COUNSELING

An oncology-trained therapist can teach you additional tools for dealing with post-medical care. Ask your doctor, medical team, or support group for names and numbers.

SUPPORT GROUP

Join a group with people who have completed medical care. Together you can process ideas for how to more easily move through anxiety, depression, and other emotions. You give and receive support and information.

EATING

Find out from your doctor about any post-treatment food restrictions, experimenting with various preparations of these. Tastes often change during medical care and stay changed for a period of time post-medical care. What tasted good before treatment may not taste good at all now. It may taste good again at some point, though. Most important, of course, is maintaining a highly nutritious diet.

EXERCISE

Every day we hear how important it is to exercise for physical and psychological wellness. Post-medical care is certainly no exception. Check with your doctor first, then "get moving" according to recommendations given to you.

SLEEPING

You may find sleep patterns are disrupted from medical care or dealing with anxious or depressed feelings. Please go to RESOURCES at the end of the book for tools focused on restorative sleep.

SUMMARY

After the magnificent celebration at the completion of cancer medical care, it is not uncommon for anxiety and depression to return. Rejoining life presents new challenges and emotional vulnerability post-cancer. Using a variety of emotional wellness tools like *triangle breathing, shifting your focus, and moving forward number-by-number* helps you go forward in this new chapter of life after cancer.

4
Outcomes—Metastasis and Recurrence

Both despair and anger often accompany recurrence of cancer and metastatic cancer. Like being in the path of a freight train, these deliver a blow that is difficult to comprehend.

Having metastatic cancer means the tumor has spread from the original location to another location in the body, often but not always to the lungs, bones, or liver. Metastatic cancer can be referred to as a chronic disease by many doctors and is usually considered incurable. Medical care is focused on managing the tumor and symptoms caused by cancer. Some patients learn they have metastatic cancer when first diagnosed.

Recurrence is similar to metastatic cancer. Local recurrence is cancer returning to where it originally began.

Distant recurrence is cancer traveling to another place in the body.

Either way, metastatic cancer or a recurrence deliver a fierce emotional slam. But you have many tools to deal with despair, anger, and other emotions.

TOOLS FOR DESPAIR AND ANGER

The Basics: Tangible items always available in your Emotional Wellness Toolbox
- This book
- A container to hold all of your materials
- Pen
- Pack of 3 x 5 index cards
- Spiral notebook
- Journal
- CDs—music
- CDs—meditation/relaxation; creative visualization; guided imagery

GIVE YOURSELF TIME
Time for comprehending new diagnosis; thoughts, feelings

TAKE CARE OF YOURSELF
Do what feels soothing

SCHEDULE A CONSULT WITH YOUR DOCTOR
Take a family member or friend with you

AFFIRMATIONS FOR EMOTIONAL WELLNESS
Helpful sparks of inspiration

WHAT WOULD A FAVORITE TEACHER ADVISE ME
Imagine talking to that one who seemed to know what to do

WHAT COULD I DO, RIGHT NOW, TO FEEL BETTER?
One action you could take to ease emotion

WHAT INSPIRED ME TODAY?
Looking for inspiration

I WAS SURPRISED WHEN….
Connecting with every day surprises

WHAT THOUGHTS DO YOU THINK MOST OF THE TIME?
Recycling self-defeating thoughts?

GETTING THROUGH CHALLENGING TIME
Segment by segment

EVALUATE WHETHER YOU ARE "RUNNING ON EMPTY"
Filling your tank

SOMETIMES ALL YOU CAN DO IS "SHOW UP"
Getting through "it" anyway

DON'T STUFF YOUR FEELINGS
You can't successfully keep them pushed down

"DELETE"
Thought stopping

TIME OUT
Take one!

FIVE THINGS YOU COULD DO TO RELAX
Take action now

LET IT GO/SHRED IT
Dumping it out

JOURNAL
Writing it down

FOCUS ON WHAT YOU CAN DO
Questions to ask yourself

CATCH YOURSELF SAYING "YES BUT"
And stop it!

SEE AN ONCOLOGY SOCIAL WORKER, PSYCHOLOGIST
Get a referral from your doctor or medical team

GO TO A SUPPORT GROUP
Get support and information about recurring and metastatic cancer

CONTINUE WITH GOOD NUTRITION
Restrictions on what to eat? Ask your doctor

CONTINUE EXERCISING
What can you do to stay active? Check with your doctor

CONTINUE GETTING RESTORATIVE SLEEP
Resources for enhancing sleep are in RESOURCES, find them in the back of this book

TOOLS 'HOW TO'

GIVE YOURSELF TIME

"Hearing" a diagnosis of metastatic cancer or recurrence requires time for absorbing, just as it did upon hearing the initial cancer diagnosis.

Allow yourself to think what you think and feel what you feel. Meet metastasis and recurrence head on. If you find your feelings or thoughts are interfering with daily functioning, call you doctor. Additionally, make an appointment with a therapist who can guide you through this challenging time.

Thoughts you may be thinking ~

Is this it?

Am I dying?

How will I get through this?

How will my family get through this?

What happens now?

Why me?

I don't want to go through it all again.

I can't handle this.

I am exhausted.

Feel what you feel. The range of feelings might find you in disbelief, or being scared, worried, overwhelmed, tired, confused, frustrated, numb, anxious, angry, depressed, nervous, shaken, shocked, outraged, betrayed, hopeless, distressed, as if you've lost control, or whatever other thoughts and feelings are swirling around you.

TAKE CARE OF YOURSELF

Giving yourself some time to do what you find relaxing and soothing is important for emotional wellness.

Go for a walk, hike, run, or swim if cleared by your doctor to do so.

Spend time with your dog or cat.

Watch your fish swim.

Hold your favorite person's hand.

Sit in the forest.

Be by the water.

Sit in your favorite chair and just *be*.

Call a friend.

Journal.

Light a candle.

SCHEDULE A CONSULT WITH YOUR DOCTOR

Take your family member or friend with you for a second pair of ears and for note taking. Learn everything you can about this new cancer including treatment options.

Make a new tab for your binder to organize new material.

AFFIRMATIONS FOR EMOTIONAL WELLNESS

Choose quotes, inspiring stories, and blog posts offering a continual supply of support. Collect and store these in your emotional wellness files, ever ready to read.

WHAT WOULD A FAVORITE TEACHER ADVISE ME

Imagine talking to that one who seemed to know what to do in various situations. What advice do you think they would offer?

Did this person have a favorite saying or quote that could help you?

WHAT COULD I DO *RIGHT NOW* TO FEEL BETTER?

What ONE action could you take to feel better right now? Just getting a drink of water, getting more comfortable in your chair, calling a friend, or looking at a magazine…anything else you can think of to comfort yourself.

WHAT *INSPIRED* ME TODAY?

Looking for inspiration helps increase your emotional wellness. Maybe it was the squirrel that dropped the nut but kept returning to the ground to pick it up. Or perhaps it was the movie you watched.

I WAS *SURPRISED* WHEN….

Like focusing on daily inspirations, looking for what surprises you on a daily basis can bring joy from unexpected sources. Perhaps someone complimented your smile, you found ten dollars in your pocket, or a friend treated you to lunch.

WHAT THOUGHTS DO YOU THINK *MOST* OF THE TIME?

Are you stuck in a negative thought pattern? Are you recycling self-defeating thoughts? Research has shown we recycle the same thoughts thousands of times a day. Thinking the same thoughts, time after time, is much like being on a hamster wheel, listening to a barrage of chatter. Become aware of what you think about and then actively choose what you *want* to think about.

GETTING THROUGH A CHALLENGING TIME SEGMENT-BY-SEGMENT

When you have cancer, it's easy to fast-forward your thinking into wondering what's going to happen. A good way to interrupt *futurizing* is to keep your thoughts in a segment-by-segment mode. When pilots fly a plane, they do not fly in a perfectly straight line from Seattle to Manhattan. They fly from Point A to Point B, then Point B to Point C, and so forth in small segments. With this tool, you do the same thing.

Since no one has all of the answers anyway, thinking too far ahead may quickly result in despair and anger.

Choose to stay focused on what's happening right now. When you get new information, focus on that.

EVALUATE WHETHER YOU ARE *RUNNING ON EMPTY*

Think about a car. It goes without saying, regardless of gas prices, if you don't fill your tank when it's empty, you won't be going anywhere. Likewise when you neglect to fill your own *psychological tank*, emotional wellness is greatly affected.

How do you keep your tank filled? How will you keep your tank filled on a continual basis? Evaluate and monitor the level of *gas* in your tank often, adding more as needed.

SOMETIMES ALL YOU CAN DO IS *SHOW UP*

Showing up may be all you can do sometimes…and that's okay. After showing up, focus on breathing long, slow, deep inhales and exhales which results in a greater sense of calm.

DON'T *STUFF* YOUR FEELINGS

People tend to do this. The problem comes when feelings erupt, and in my experience, they will. You can keep them pushed down only so long. *Feel what you feel,* acknowledge what you feel, then choose and carry out a positive, beneficial action.

"DELETE"

On a 3 x 5 card write down one thought that is keeping you emotionally stirred up—

"I just don't know what to do about….," then close your eyes and imagine writing that exact thought on the computer. Imagine highlighting the thought and pushing *delete*. (If the computer is handy, do type out the thought and delete it).

Leave the thought deleted. Refuse to start thinking it all over again. Instead, try active problem solving.

Write down what you are solving at the top of your spiral notebook. Then brainstorm ways to solve it thinking of every possible solution you can. Do not leave anything out even if the solution seems far-fetched. When you have a list of solutions, choose one and follow through taking action.

If you don't feel satisfied with the outcome of this exercise, perhaps talking it over with a therapist, a friend, or a family member would be helpful. What isn't helpful is keeping yourself emotionally stirred up. Let go and actively find a solution.

TIME OUT

Take a time out from despair and anger. Imagine putting these emotions in a box beside you. Then take needed time for relaxing or for doing something you want to accomplish without these emotions. They will wait in the box until your time out is over.

FIVE THINGS YOU COULD DO TO RELAX

In your spiral notebook, at the top of the page write:

FIVE THINGS I COULD DO TO RELAX OR FEEL LESS STRESSED IN FIVE MINUTES

One third from the top of the page write:

FIVE THINGS I COULD DO TO RELAX OR FEEL LESS STRESSED IN FIFTEEN MINUTES

Two thirds from the top of the page write:

FIVE THINGS I COULD DO TO RELAX OR FEEL LESS STRESSED IN THIRTY MINUTES

Ideas for five minutes:

- Take some deep breaths
- Write down an affirmation ten times
- Read a helpful affirmation or quote ten times
- Look outside at the squirrel, the flowers, the dog strolling by

Ideas for fifteen minutes:

- Listen to your favorite music
- Triangle Breathing (see triangle breathing tool in Chapter 1)
- Write soothing thoughts in your journal
- Encourage yourself with self talk (see self-talk tool in Chapter 2)

Ideas for thirty minutes

- Eat something you enjoy
- Watch a favorite TV show
- Take a power nap
- Quiet my mind by taking a time out (see time out tool in Chapter 4)

Then get three 3 x 5 cards and at the top of the first card write Five Things I Can Do To Relax For Five Minutes; at the top of the second card write Five Things I Can Do To Relax For Fifteen Minutes; and at the top of the third card, write Five Things I Can Do To Relax for Thirty Minutes.

List each of your five relaxation ideas under the appropriate time frame. Carry these cards with you in your purse, briefcase, or folder where you have easy access to them. When you find yourself getting antsy, feeling despair, or feeling angry, use these cards to help you relax. You may find this tool especially helpful while in an office waiting room, while waiting for a phone call, or when you need a break.

LET IT GO/SHRED IT

In her book, *The Artist's Way*, Julia Cameron discusses the exercise of writing three pages of thoughts and feelings each morning before you do anything else. This is an excellent tool for *dumping out* thoughts and feelings.

Many people I work with are very hesitant to use this tool because they are concerned someone will find and read what they write down. To alleviate this concern, I suggest shredding their pages after completing them. The tool becomes even more powerful when focusing on *letting go* of troublesome thoughts and feelings as the papers are shredded.

JOURNAL

Journaling, on the other hand, is a progression of thoughts and feelings you write down as desired. Some people find rereading what they have written very helpful.

A related tool is the video journal. If you have a newer model computer, the camera is built in. Film yourself discussing thoughts and feelings.

FOCUS ON WHAT YOU *CAN* DO

Sometimes, you may find yourself caught up in swirling emotion that just keeps on swirling, keeping you from moving forward. Try some problem solving questions.

Write down in your spiral notebook a situation bothering you. Then write down and answer the questions:

How can I _____?

What can I _____?

You are now putting your focus on a specific action you can take.

CATCH YOURSELF SAYING "YES, BUT" AND *STOP IT*

When you are seeking a solution to a problem, sometimes a solution comes to mind or another person offers a suggestion. Instead of considering the solution, you say

"Yes, but….I can't."

"Yes, but it won't work out because….."

"Yes, but I don't have time to…."

"Yes, but I don't have money for…"

In effect, when you immediately look for the negatives, you are erasing a possible solution before giving it full and fair consideration.

Decide instead to take the thought or suggestion and think it through, looking for whether any or part of it could, in fact, offer a solution.

SEE AN ONCOLOGY SOCIAL WORKER OR PSYCHOLOGIST

Ask your doctor and medical team for a referral and then make an appointment. Get help for moving forward emotionally with recurring and metastatic cancer.

GO TO A SUPPORT GROUP

Seek out a support group for boosting emotional wellness for people coping with metastatic or recurrent cancer.

CONTINUE WITH GOOD NUTRITION

Learn from your doctor what foods you can eat now. Are there any restrictions? If available, ask your doctor for a referral to a dietician.

CONTINUE EXERCISING

What can you do to stay active? Ask your doctor what exercises you can do now and then follow through.

CONTINUE GETTING RESTORATIVE SLEEP

Getting *good sleep* is essential for the body and for emotional wellness. Please go to the end of the book in the section on RESOURCES for a list of CD's to enhance sleep.

SUMMARY

Being diagnosed with metastatic cancer or recurring cancer can find you coping with significant anger and despair. Time is needed to comprehend this news and to emotionally move forward through the diagnosis. Using emotional wellness tools like *time out, one action you could take right now, and getting through segment-by-segment* will help you meet the challenge to emotional wellness arising from a diagnosis of metastatic or recurrent cancer.

5
Outcomes—Grieving

When a diagnosis is made indicating treatment will no longer be helpful, anticipatory grief begins. Anticipatory grief is defined by David Kessler as "the beginning of the end in our minds. We now operate in two worlds; the safe world that we are used to and the unsafe world where a loved one might die. We feel that sadness and the unconscious need to prepare our psyche." (Kessler 2000, 2012)

Anticipatory grief can be a solitary, internal process marked by an unwillingness to verbalize feelings about the coming loss. Patients, family members, friends, and caregivers all usually experience anticipatory grief.

Grieving after the actual death of a loved one is generally experienced differently by each person. Research has identified common emotional responses such as anger, denial, and depression. What was once believed to be a relatively linear process of stages based on elapsed time from death, grieving is now understood by many researchers as a nonlinear process with elements of unpredictability regarding the length of time any one person may need to experience the loss.

Anticipatory grief and grieving are not easy. It is terribly difficult to think about *letting go* before death and to *let go* of the person you love when death comes. Yet few lives are untouched by profound loss. Grieving for the loved ones who die is part of the human condition.

Gratefully, we have systems in place to help cope with the inevitable. These include both palliative care and hospice care, which incorporate a team of doctors, nurses, social workers, and other medical caregivers into an approach centering on the comfortable care of patients at the end-stages of disease.

Palliative Care and Hospice Care

Confusion regarding the definitions of palliative care and hospice care is widespread. Both center on the patient's quality of life, with a focus on symptom and pain management. Both address adjustment concerns related to cancer and dealing with death and dying.

Palliative care and hospice care differ in both medical treatment and when a patient can qualify for care. In palliative care, medical treatment can continue for as long as is needed and does not require a terminal prognosis. For hospice, the patient has a terminal prognosis with a life expectancy of six months or less. Additionally, medical treatment has been determined to no longer be of benefit, and pain management takes center stage.

Hospice is a choice. For patients with cancer, the patient, family members, and caregivers decide whether to utilize hospice. The medical care team can be very helpful with information and advice when making the decision about whether to go with hospice care.

While hospice care begins when curative medical care ends, palliative care is often linked with medical care as cancer progresses. It is currently becoming more prevalent, starting earlier in the course of disease and focusing on the patient's quality of life.

TOOLS FOR ANTICIPATORY GRIEF AND GRIEVING

The Basics: Tangible items always available in your Emotional Wellness Toolbox
- This book
- A container to hold all of your materials
- Pen

- Pack of 3 x 5 index cards
- Spiral notebook
- Journal
- CDs—music
- CDs—meditation/relaxation; creative visualization; guided imagery

TIME STOPS
What to do now

QUESTIONS TO ASK YOURSELF
Answers guide you through

ADVANCED DIRECTIVES
Tool for helping you clarify

FLOWING WITH GRIEF
Moving through grief

CONVERSATION WITH YOURSELF
It's okay to feel.....

LOOKING FOR A SMILE
How to find one

TAKING CARE TO TAKE CARE OF YOU
Moments matter

"CALLING OUT" GRIEF
Gaining insight

TAKE A GRIEF BREAK
Pause it

FIND A THEME SONG
Encouraging words

ONE STEP AT A TIME
Tight Rope Walking

TLC YOURSELF
Five things you can do

HAVE CONVERSATIONS
Talk, talk, talk

SEND YOURSELF A CARD
Soothing words

SCHEDULING YOUR TIME
Structure is good

TALK WITH YOUR DOCTOR IF
Grief is interfering with normal functioning

SEE AN ONCOLOGY SOCIAL WORKER, PSYCHOLOGIST
Get a referral from your doctor or medical team

GO TO A SUPPORT GROUP
Grief groups are available

GOOD NUTRITION
Eat nutritiously

EXERCISING
What can you do to stay active? Check with your doctor

RESTORATIVE SLEEP
Resources for enhancing sleep are in RESOURCES, find them
in the back of this book

TOOLS 'HOW TO'

TIME STOPS

Both anticipatory grief and grieving are *time stopping*. Your attention is focused on *right now, up front, this can't be happening/ this is happening.* Give yourself that time to just be distracted. You may want to talk with your boss, your family, your teachers, and whoever else is in your daily life so they understand your distress.

Take time to just *be* with your grief. Cry, scream, get mad, kick the soccer ball, take a hot shower, punch the punching bag, journal, fret, get coffee with a friend, pet the dog and the cat, paint a picture, go fishing, look at the stars, plant some flowers, light a candle, send yourself some flowers, walk in nature, or do whatever else that help as long as it is not harmful to yourself or others.

QUESTIONS TO ASK YOURSELF

Ask and answer these questions:

What are my thoughts and feelings about death and dying?

How will I take care of myself physically, emotionally, and spiritually while dying takes place?

How can I best support my loved one during this time?

What are my thoughts and feelings about hospice care?

How will I say goodbye to my beloved? When will I say goodbye?

Do I have anything that "needs" to be resolved with my loved one? If so, do I resolve it with that person or do I resolve it in another way such as talking with a psychotherapist, writing a letter (does not get sent), etc.

ADVANCED DIRECTIVES

Advanced directives are important documents for letting your doctor know what medical care you want to have or not have when death is at hand. It is necessary to complete these before they are needed. Since states vary on how they are managed, be certain you know what your state requires for advanced directives. Please see RESOURCES at the end of the book.

FLOWING WITH GRIEF

You cannot run away from grief and grieving. It is a normal emotional process and is necessary to go through. You may find yourself crying one minute, angry the next, and deciding you are just fine in the next (though you don't really feel just fine). Expect this. It's all part of normal grieving.

CONVERSATION WITH YOURSELF

Have a conversation with yourself, aloud if you are alone. Let yourself know it is okay to feel what you feel. Giving yourself permission to grieve and acknowledging what you feel goes a long way to help you move through your feelings. Trying to *stuff* your grief and be stoic doesn't work as feelings can only be pushed down temporarily. They will surface.

LOOKING FOR A SMILE

Grief and smiles do not often go hand-in-hand. Yet, taking a bit of time to smile is helpful for lightening the weight of grief. Some people feel guilty when they smile while going through their sadness, but it's okay to smile. *What one thing could you find right now to smile about?*

TAKING CARE TO TAKE CARE OF YOU

Find moments to soothe yourself. What could you do right now for you? You could treat yourself to an ice cream cone, watch the little boy swing at the park, wake up early to see the sunrise, or something else. Get a 3 x 5 card and write down the day and date at the top. Then, each day keep track of what you are doing for yourself. Write down at least two things each day.

CALLING OUT GRIEF

Find a way to learn more about your grief. For example could you draw a picture of it or make up a poem about it? Could you write an article or a story about grief? While this may be the last thing you feel like doing, when you just do it anyway, surprising insight can surface.

TAKE A GRIEF BREAK

While feeling and experiencing your grief is essential to moving through it, taking a break is okay too. Choose a comfortable amount of time and set your timer or watch accordingly. Then, take just that period of time to do something else, an activity unrelated to grieving.

FIND A THEME SONG

Choose a song that moves you, encourages you, and offers strength. Listen to it. Sing it! Write the words down on a 3 x 5 card. Music can go a long way to soothe the sadness of grieving.

ONE STEP AT A TIME

Think of a tightrope walker to help you move forward. A tightrope walker must move ever so slowly forward. If she looks down falling is a real possibility. If she looks too far left or too far right falling is a real possibility, or if she looks too far across, hurrying a bit to get to the other side in order to get off the tightrope, falling is a real possibility. Grieving is like that. Grieving takes its own time. It can't be rushed or hurried.

TLC YOURSELF

Give yourself some TLC—some Tender Loving Care. This is a good thing to keep in mind throughout grieving. Grieving calls for being especially gentle and loving with yourself, continually finding ways to soothe and ease the emotions you are experiencing. Keep a running list in your spiral notebook of ways to *TLC Yourself.* Refer to it often for ideas.

HAVE CONVERSATIONS

It is okay to talk about your grief with others. Sometimes hearing yourself talk about it can offer insight and direction. Additionally, the listener may be able to offer helpful suggestions. Actively choose people to talk with about your grief who will be supportive.

SEND YOURSELF A CARD

Go to the store, pick out a beautiful card, and send it to yourself. Find a card with encouraging, supportive words and then write some of your own. Mail it to yourself. Enjoy opening your card and put it in a place where you will see it often.

SCHEDULING YOUR TIME

While you may not feel much like any kind of schedule or routine when you are grieving, try to keep some semblance of one. This is certainly not the time to be rigid with yourself, but having some structure can give you back a sense of being in control and help move you forward.

GO SEE YOUR DOCTOR

If grieving is interfering with functioning in your activities of daily life, schedule a time with your doctor. Sometimes grief can be so deep and intense that medical intervention is needed.

SEE AN ONCOLOGY SOCIAL WORKER, PSYCHOLOGIST

Going to see a therapist while grieving can be of great benefit. Being *heard* is very soothing. In addition, she can offer guidance for continuing to move through grief.

GO TO A SUPPORT GROUP

Support groups for those grieving or grappling with anticipatory grief are available. Being around others who are experiencing similar emotions and issues can offer great support.

GOOD NUTRITION

Sometimes people who are grieving find that they have no appetite while others find themselves continually eating. Neither of these are good choices. Instead, pay particular attention to eating nutritiously and to choosing appropriate quantities.

EXERCISING

With your doctor's go ahead, continue to stay as active as you can. Clearly, exercise helps bring balance and ease to emotions.

RESTORATIVE SLEEP

Resources for enhancing sleep are in RESOURCES at the end of the book.

SUMMARY

Grief, whether it arises from the anticipation of a loss or from the actual loss, is emotionally challenging. While researchers have identified common emotional responses, people grieve differently and for various amounts of time.

Of *most* importance is to give yourself the time and space to go through the grieving process as you need to experience it, without being hurried or told that "…it's been long enough."

6
Outcomes—Loss

Emotional wellness returns after grieving over your loss, sometimes in *roller coaster* fashion. That is, you may find yourself feeling good in the morning and moving easily through routine activities, but sad in the afternoon and finding it difficult to interact and stay engaged with people. This is normal. Life after loss is never the same. Anything can instantly remind you of the person you have lost. Grieving is a process that happens slowly, where emotions only become soothed or balanced after sufficient time to assimilate your loss has passed.

Emotional wellness in this context is determined by you. You know when you are feeling relaxed inside, handling daily tasks, and participating easily within relationships. It is a feeling you cannot force—grieving takes its own time. But emotional wellness will return and you will move forward through your grief. If at any time you are concerned about the intensity of your feelings, or if your emotions are interfering with daily functioning, talk with your doctor or counselor.

TOOLS FOR EMOTIONAL WELLNESS AND LOSS

The Basics: Tangible items always available in your Emotional Wellness Toolbox
- This book
- A container to hold all of your materials
- Pen
- Pack of 3 x 5 index cards
- Spiral notebook
- Journal
- CDs—music
- CDs—meditation/relaxation; creative visualization; guided imagery

MANAGING LOSS
Memories, Birthdays, Anniversaries

FEELING GUILTY?
Sometimes you do

SOOTHING SELF
Emotional balm

WHAT ARE THE GIFTS?
Good things

HOW COULD I?
Move yourself forward quickly

WHAT HELPED ME TODAY?
Insight for tomorrow

SMILES?
Bring them on

MAGNIFY WELLBEING
How to expand it

ONE THING IN YOUR POCKET
Take it with you

THE OKAY METER
Moving forward on it

HELIUM BALLOONS
Concern be gone

ASK YOURSELF WHY NOT?
Then follow through

HOLD YOUR OWN HAND
Showing up for yourself

SHRINK IT
Contracting a thought or feeling

SEE AN ONCOLOGY SOCIAL WORKER, PSYCHOLOGIST
Get a referral from your doctor or medical team

CONTINUE WITH GOOD NUTRITION
Enhances emotional wellness

CONTINUE EXERCISING

CONTINUE GETTING RESTORATIVE SLEEP
Resources for enhancing sleep can be found in the back of
this book

TOOLS 'HOW TO'

MANAGING LOSS

Emotional wellness does not mean you will no longer feel emotion from memories you have or when birthdays and anniversaries occur. In fact, emotions often intensify as you remember your loved one. Sometimes you may be caught off guard, one minute you're feeling just fine, the next crying when you think about the time…..

Birthdays and anniversaries are known for stirring up emotions as you remember these special times shared with your loved one. Expect this and set time aside to acknowledge the occasion.

It is normal to feel yourself move back into grieving when you think about memories or special celebration days. Be easy with yourself and *lean into* the emotion allowing yourself to feel what you feel. Gradually these feelings will subside and emotional wellness will return.

FEELING GUILTY?

As you begin new relationships, you may find yourself feeling guilty or feeling concerned about betraying the relationship you had with your loved one. This is a normal feeling. What would your loved one say to you? Would your loved one want you to be happy, to move forward, to establish new connections with life as it is now?

SOOTHING YOURSELF

What is your emotional balm? What is it you do for yourself to enhance emotional wellbeing? Write these down in your spiral notebook and use them for soothing. You might also want to take your list, rewriting it on 3 x 5 cards, one item per card. Then, turn them over so you can't see the writing, shuffle, and pick one to do for yourself.

WHAT ARE THE GIFTS?

As the "rawness" of loss heals, spend some time focusing on the many good things in your life. Start a list in your spiral notebook. Continue adding daily to your list, reflecting on these. You may want to use a journal for recording your thoughts about the gifts. Some people have a dedicated gratitude journal.

HOW COULD I?

After loss, sometimes it's difficult to motivate yourself to take on new relationships or new activities. You can keep yourself from moving forward by believing too much effort is involved.

Try thinking of something you would like to accomplish and write it down at the top of a page in your spiral notebook. Then think of one tiny thing you could do moving you in the direction of accomplishing that thing. One tiny action moves you closer; a string of tiny actions gets you where you want to go.

WHAT *HELPED* ME TODAY?

Find a time each day to reflect on what is helping you move forward, enhancing your emotional wellness. Keep a list of these tools in your spiral notebook. Read them often and add to them.

SMILES

What brings a smile to you?

Think it.

Do it.

Watch it.

Be it.

Create it.

Look at a picture of it.

Listen to it.

Paint it.

Smell it.

Write it.

Touch it.

Gather it.

Cook it.

MAGNIFY EMOTIONAL WELLNESS

When you focus on emotional wellness you will find yourself feeling more emotionally well since what we focus on expands. This tool involves "playing with" emotional wellness.

Imagine you are completely filled with emotional wellness. How do you feel? Write a letter to yourself explaining in detail what it's like to feel emotionally well.

Could you make up a song about it? Or, could you sing a song you know that represents emotional wellness for you? What about creating something that represents emotional wellness. Maybe you will sculpt clay, paint, carve, build, paint, plant, etc. something meaningful.

ONE THING IN YOUR POCKET

Choose one thing you can keep in your pocket symbolizing peace, courage, or anything else helpful to you. You might choose a favorite coin, a small heart, a favorite fortune from a fortune cookie, or you may want to create something.

Whatever you choose, each time you take the small object out to look at it, associate it with peace, courage, or what is helpful for you.

THE OKAY METER

In your imagination or on a piece of paper in your spiral notebook, create a round circle with a dial. Circle numbers one through ten around the dial. One is a low rating on the OK meter indicating things are not feeling OK inside. Ten is a high rating, indicating you are feeling very OK, fabulous OK. Where are you on the OK meter? Check in with yourself frequently. Maybe right now you are coming in as a 3. Could you raise it to 4, 5, or an 8? How would you do that? Think of specific actions you could take right now to push the number higher.

HELIUM BALLOON

Visualize psychologically *letting go* of an issue that is troublesome to you. Imagine writing down what's bothering you on a 3 x 5 card, inserting the folded card into a helium balloon, and watching the balloon carry the concern away. You can also use this tool for worry, unfounded fear, being overwhelmed, anxiety, or any other unwanted emotion.

ASK YOURSELF WHY NOT?

Why not go out for coffee?

Why not check into that exercise program?

Why not sign up for the hike?

Why not take the class?

Why not get a puppy?

Why not......?

Sometimes after loss, you may need a nudge to help yourself get going. *Why not?* is a simple question and, when answered, spurs action.

HOLD YOUR OWN HAND

Most of us are fortunate to have two hands and can do this. Holding your own hand can be very soothing when you think about it in this way.

SHRINK IT

If you are feeling scared, worried, or something similar, imagine that feeling in the palm of your hand. See if you can shrink that feeling to a smaller form, and then gently blow it off your palm. Let the feeling go.

MAKE AN APPOINTMENT WITH AN ONCOLOGY COUNSELOR

Even when you've moved from loss to emotional wellness, you still can benefit from seeing a therapist. An oncology social worker or psychologist can assist you with tools for boosting and maintaining emotional wellness.

CONTINUE WITH GOOD NUTRITION

Eating well naturally enhances emotional wellness. You might want to get creative trying some new recipes or tasting some new foods. Why not?

CONTINUE EXERCISING

Exercising is well known for releasing chemicals that help to maximize emotional wellness.

CONTINUE GETTING RESTORATIVE SLEEP

Restorative sleep is clearly important for amplifying emotional wellness. Please see RESOURCES at the end of this book suggested CD's focused on getting restorative sleep.

SUMMARY

Moving through loss restores you to emotional wellness in roller coaster fashion. That is, one minute you might feel good and the next you may return to grief and be overwhelmed with sadness. This is normal. Emotional wellness continues to expand in your life as you assimilate the loss of your loved one. Key emotional tools include learning how to cope with important dates, memories, and beginning new relationships.

Conclusion

Cancer and emotional wellness must go hand in hand. Much attention is paid to medical treatment and now, thankfully, many of us "get" the paramount role emotions figure into the cancer arena.

Cancer undeniably affects everyone in the patient's circle of care: spouse/partner, family members, caregivers and friends. Much like trying to piece together a puzzle having pieces of other puzzles tossed in, moving through cancer is at best a journey of continually changing unknowns.

Emotional and psychological wellbeing can accompany you, if you choose to take that route. It is a choice, however challenging. It is easy to feel a loss of control with changing cancer demands, but you can powerfully effect how you go through cancer by making this choice.

An abundance of strategies and tools are offered here for you to take with you on the cancer voyage. They are specifically designed to be easy, effective, and require little of the precious time and energy you have when dealing with cancer.

These strategies and tools are products of my work as a psychotherapist with cancer patients, their loved ones and others in their circle of care. The tools are constantly evolving so I would like to hear from you about your cancer experience. Tell me which tools are working for you, and tell me if you have suggestions for new tools. Please let me know by e-mailing me at: niki@canceremotionalwellbeing.com.

Meanwhile, I wish for you peace in the midst of the turmoil that often accompanies cancer. Journey calmly and confidently, one step at a time, through these unknown paths while deeply cherishing and caring for your own emotional wellness.

Appendix A
Resources

In this appendix, you will find a variety of resources to help you explore all aspects of emotional wellness in more depth. Resources include books, magazines, websites, and CDs.

BOOKS

Cameron, L. (1992). *The Artist's Way.* NY: Penguin Putnam.

Carr, K. (2008). *Crazy Sexy Cancer Survivor.* Guilford, CT: Morris.

Kris has written about her experiences as a survivor. She includes many tips for moving forward when you are re-joining daily life as I discussed in Chapter 3. For example, on page 90, Kris discusses writing down 10 things you'd like to try now and on page 102, she suggests keeping a gratitude journal.

Carr, K. (2007). *Crazy sexy cancer tips.* Guilford, CT: Morris. Writing about her experience of cancer, Kris offers a variety of tips for coping with cancer. Additionally, she profiles other women dealing with various kinds of cancer. For example, tip 44 on page 91 suggests, "doing what makes you feel better and offers hope". This book is particularly good for young women.

Grant, B., Block, A., Hamilton, K., & Thomson, C. (2010). *American Cancer Society Complete Nutrition for Cancer Survivors*. Atlanta: American Cancer Society.

As we discussed eating well is very important throughout cancer (Chapters 1-6). You will find this book a good, comprehensive resource for nutrition covering all stages of cancer and beyond. It tackles various nutrition dilemmas such as challenges with eating during treatment.

Siegel, B. (2011). *A Book of Miracles: Inspiring true stories of healing gratitude, and love*. Novato: New Wave Library.

Love, compassion, inspiration, and healing stories are woven together from surgeon Bernie's time with his patients. An excellent resource for emotional support.

Siegel, B. (2003). *365 Prescriptions for the Soul: Daily messages of inspiration, hope and love*. Novato: New World Library.

Bernie takes each day and offers a meditation filled with inspiration, hope, humor and empowerment. Another excellent resource for emotional support.

Siegel, B. (1998). ***Love, Medicine and Miracles: Lessons learned about self-healing from a surgeon's experience with exceptional patients.*** New York: HarperPerrenial.

Through steady listening and empathy with his patients, surgeon Bernie Siegel helped patients feel "heard" and "loved" in their journey. Cancer patients I worked with continually discussed how vital being listened to is. This book offers much encouragement and empowerment.

Silver, J. ed. (2009). ***What Helped Het Me Through: Cancer survivors share wisdom and hope.*** Atlanta: American Cancer Society. This book includes stories of cancer survivors and celebrity cancer survivors exploring how they dealt with various issues including their emotions.

As we discussed throughout Emotional Wellness, counseling with a trained oncology therapist can be very helpful, wherever you are in the cancer journey. In Chapter 14 titled "What

Helped Me Heal," survivors talk about their experiences with counseling.

MAGAZINES

Cancer Today
(http://www.cancertodaymag.org/Pages/default.aspx)

This magazine offers a variety of articles based on nutrition, exercise, and communication. On the home page, click on "Living With Cancer" and you will find useful information supplementing the emotional tools you have read about it in this book.

Coping with Cancer
(http://copingmag.com/cwc/)

Rejoining daily life can be very challenging when cancer treatment is over (Chapter 3). A current featured article deals with how to move forward offering helpful suggestions. One powerful tool for coping with anger and despair (Chapter 4) is keeping a file of inspiring quotes and stories. On the home page under the tab "Inspiration" by clicking "Words of Inspiration" you will find words of support you can collect for your emotional tool file.

Cure Today

(http://www.curetoday.com)

On the home page click on "Cancer Journey" and find listed the steps of cancer (Chapter 1-6) including diagnosis, treatment, post treatment, metastatic cancer, and survivorship. You will find easy and effective tools for helping you move forward emotionally such as "meditation tips" (Chapter 1 and 3).

CDs

How to Meditate with Pema Chodron: A Practical Guide to Making Friends with Your Mind (Audiobook, Unabridged) (Audio CD) Pema Chodron (Author). This set of CD's is particularly useful for understanding how powerful meditation is and most helpful when you've had some experience meditating. It is not focused on specific guided meditations.

Meditation for Beginners: 10th-Anniversary Edition (Abridged, Audiobook) (Audio CD) Jack Kornfield (Author).

You will find this CD a good source for learning how to meditate. Jack uses storytelling providing much insight into meditation and guides you through meditations.

A Meditation to Help You with Healthful Sleep (Audiobook) (Audio CD) Belleruth Naparstek (Author).

You will find Belleruth's voice soothing as she uses guided imagery to help you relax into sleep. After she has finished the meditation, music continues to further promote sleep.

A Meditation to Help You Relieve Depression
(Audiobook) (Audio CD) Belleruth Naparstek (Author).

This CD is NOT a substitute for counseling or medication, if needed for depression. It is a good tool to use in conjunction with counseling and medication if depression is not interfering with your daily functioning.

Wholesome Relaxation (Audiobook) (Audio CD) Julie Lusk (Author).

Incorporating soothing and easy calming exercises, boosted with affirmations and guided imagery, Julie helps you maximize relaxation skills. This is a good CD to have in your emotional toolbox.

WEBSITES

American Cancer Society

(http://www.cancer.org)

Specific information is what you will want throughout cancer. You can call (1-800-227-2345) getting information on various cancer topics such as parenting, emotional support, and financial concerns, in addition to specific information about cancer, research, and treatment. This website is directed to cancer patients, family members and caregivers.

Cancer Support Community

(http://www.cancersupportcommunity.org)

Create your own webpage on this site which allows you to keep your friends and family posted on how you're doing, allows friends and family to send you messages, allows you to add pictures and quotes, and allows other features. On the home page, click on create a webpage to get started. Think of this as an online journal, an important tool to add to your emotional toolbox.

LiveStrong

(http://www.livestrong.org)

As we discussed in Chapters 5 and 6 grief and loss are not easy to deal with. The LiveStrong website has a useful list of topics cancer survivors in particular may be faced with including physical losses, emotional losses, social and relationship losses, and financial losses. On the home page click "Get Help" then under "Learn About Cancer" click on "Emotional Effects", selecting "Grief and Loss". The lists provide validation of many things you may be feeling.

National Cancer Institute

(http://www.cancer.gov)

One of the strongest emotions challenging you when you are first diagnosed with cancer is anxiety. As we discussed in Chapter One, the National Cancer Institute website links anxiety to pain, sleep problems, nausea and vomiting. This site has excellent information on different types of cancer (click the "Types of Cancer" link on the homepage), as well as ways to cope with cancer (click "Cancer Topics" on the homepage). Their easy to understand, yet comprehensive explanations and suggestions will help you on your healing journey.

National Coalition for Cancer Survivorship

(http://www.canceradvocacy.org)

When you are diagnosed with cancer, common emotional responses are anxiety and depression, (Chapters 1, 2, and 3). Not only is it difficult to "wrap your own mind" around having cancer, telling people about your cancer adds to emotional distress. This website provides a good tool for talking about cancer with your family, friends, doctor, and employer. On the homepage click on "Living with Cancer", then click on "How to Talk About Cancer".

University of Maryland, Marlene and Stewart Greenebaum Cancer Center

(http://www.umgcc.org)

This is another excellent resource for anxiety and depression, (Chapters 1,2, and 3). On the home page, under "Patients and Families", click on "Information for Patients", then under "Cancer Topics" on the left side of the page, click on "Adjustment to Cancer: Anxiety and Distress". An additional resource under "Cancer Topics" is "Communication in Cancer Care". As discussed in each of the chapters in Emotional wellness, The Other Half of Treating Cancer, communication is an essential tool throughout all of cancer.

MD Anderson Cancer Center

(http://www.mdanderson.org)

This website provides good supplemental information on important topics such as nutrition, dealing with stress, and how to quit smoking. On the home page, go down to the bottom of the page, and click on "Focused on Health".

Appendix B
Citations

In this appendix, you will find citations from the scientific literature allowing you to explore ideas presented in the book in more technical depth.

Beatriz RV; Bamier PO; Bayon C; Palao A; Torres G; Hospital A; Guillermo B; Diegues M; Liria AF. *Differences in depressed oncologic patients' narratives after receiving two different therapeutic interventions for depression: a qualitative study.* Psycho-Oncology 2012;21(12) 1292-1298.

Brown LF; Kroenke K. *Cancer-related fatigue and its associations with depression and anxiety: A systematic review.* Psychosomatics 2009;50(5)440-447.

Cancer patients need care for anxiety (11/10). Retrieved from http://psychcentral.com/news/2010/11/11/cancer-patients-need-care-for-anxiety/20789.html

Jacobsen PB; Jim HS. *Psychosocial interventions for anxiety and depression in adult cancer patients: achievements and challenges.* CA: A Cancer Journal for Clinicians 2008;58(4)214-230.

National Cancer Institute, Washington, D.C. *Adjustment to Cancer: Anxiety and Distress* (PDQ®) http://www.cancer.gov/cancertopics/pdq/supportivecare/adjustment/Patient

NCI dictionary of terms. Retrieved from http://www.cancer.gov/dictionary?cdrid=430405

Ott MJ; Norris RL; Bauer-Wu SM. *Mindfulness meditation for oncology patients: A discussion and critical review.* Integrative Cancer Therapies 2006;5(2):98-108.

Depression (11/12). Retrieved from http://www.cancer.gov/cancertopics/pdq/supportivecare/depression/Patient

Depression and Cancer (12/10). Retrieved from http://www.hopkinsmedicine.org/kimmel_cancer_center/_downloads/patient_info/Depression and Cancer.pdf

Depression (3/11). Retrieved from http://www.cancer.org/treatment/treatmentsandsideeffects/physicalsideeffects/dealingwithsymptomsathome/caring-for-the-patient-with-cancer-at-home-depression

Cancer and Depression: When to be Concerned (11/10). Retrieved from http://www.mayoclinic.com/health/cancer-and-depression/MY01567

Depression and Anxiety (10/12). Retrieved from http://www.cancer.net/coping/emotional-and-physical-matters/depression-and-anxiety

Zucca AC; Boyes AW; Lecathelinals C; Afaf G. *Life is precious and I'm making the best of it: coping strategies of long-term cancer survivors.* Psycho-Oncology 2010;19(12)1268-1276.

Dealing with Cancer Recurrence (5/10). Retrieved from http://www.cancer.net/all-about-cancer/treating-cancer/dealing-cancer-recurrence

Krikorian A; Limonero JT; Mate J. *Suffering and distress at the end of life.* Psycho-Oncology. 2012;21(8) 799-808.

Metastatic Cancer (5/11). Retrieved from http://www.cancer.gov/cancertopics/factsheet/Sites-Types/metastatic

When Cancer Returns: How to Cope with Cancer Recurrence (2/11).

Retrieved from
http://www.mayoclinic.com/health/cancer/CA00050

Advance Directives (11/12). Retrieved from
http://www.nlm.nih.gov/medlineplus/advancedirectives.html

Casarett DJ; Quill TE. *"I'm not ready for hospice":
strategies for timely and effective hospice discussions.*
Annals of Internal Medicine 2007; 146(6)443-449.

Johansson A; Grimby A. *Anticipatory grief among close
relatives of patients in hospice and palliative wards.*
American Journal of Hospice and Palliative Medicine
2012;29(2)134-138.

Kubler-Ross E; Kessler D. *On grief and grieving: finding
the meaning of grief through the five stages of loss* (2005).
New York: Scribner.

Kessler D. *On grief and grieving: frequently asked
questions on grief and grieving.*
http://grief.com/questions-answers/on-grief-grieving/

Smith TJ. *Palliative care for oncology patients* (11/12). Retrieved from http://www.cancernetwork.com/nurses/content/article/1016 5/2111593

Types of Grief Reactions (6/11). Retrieved from http://www.cancer.gov/cancertopics/pdq/supportivecare/be reavement/Patient/

Dumont I; Dumont S; Mongeau S. *End-of-life care and the grieving process: family caregivers who have experienced the loss of a terminal-phase cancer patient.* Qualitative Health Research 2008;18(8)1049-1061.

Phillips LR; Reed PG. *Into the abyss of someone else's dying, the voice of the end-of-life caregivers.* Clinical Nursing Research 2009;18(1)80-97.

Ward-Griffin C; McWilliam CL; Oudshoorn A. *Relational experiences of family caregivers providing home-based end-of-life care.* Journal of Family Nursing 2012;18(4)491-516.

Index

About the Author

Niki Barr, PhD, founded a pioneering psychotherapy practice dedicated to working with cancer patients in all stages of cancer, along with their family members, caregivers and friends. In *Emotional Wellness: The Other Half of Treating Cancer*, she describes an Emotional Wellness Toolbox filled with strategies and tools to help cancer patients and those who care for them manage the journey through cancer with confidence and calm. In addition to her active psychotherapy practice, Dr. Barr is also a dynamic and popular speaker, sharing her insights with cancer patients and clinicians across the nation.

CPSIA information can be obtained at www.ICGtesting.com
Printed in the USA
LVOW102105080413

328040LV00004B/9/P